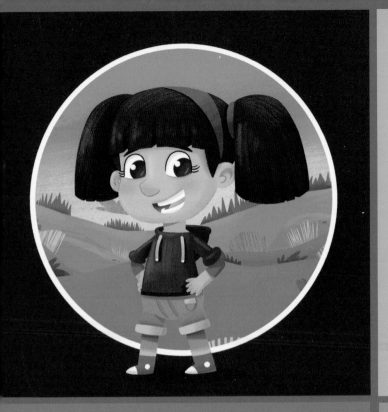

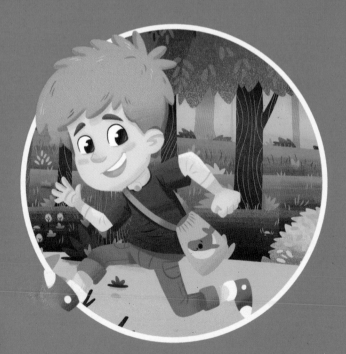

The abilities in me

This book is dedicated to George Hall, age 8 with a Tracheostomy.

First edition June 2020

Published by The Abilities In Me
Written by Gemma Keir
Illustrations copyright © 2020 by Adam Walker-Parker
Edited by Claire Bunyan and Emma Lusty

ISBN Paperback: 9798674992721

First printed in the United Kingdom, 2020

www.theabilitiesinme.com

The abilities in me

Tracheostomy

Written by Gemma Keir
Illustrated by Adam Walker-Parker

One day I visited the hospital,
as I needed surgery.

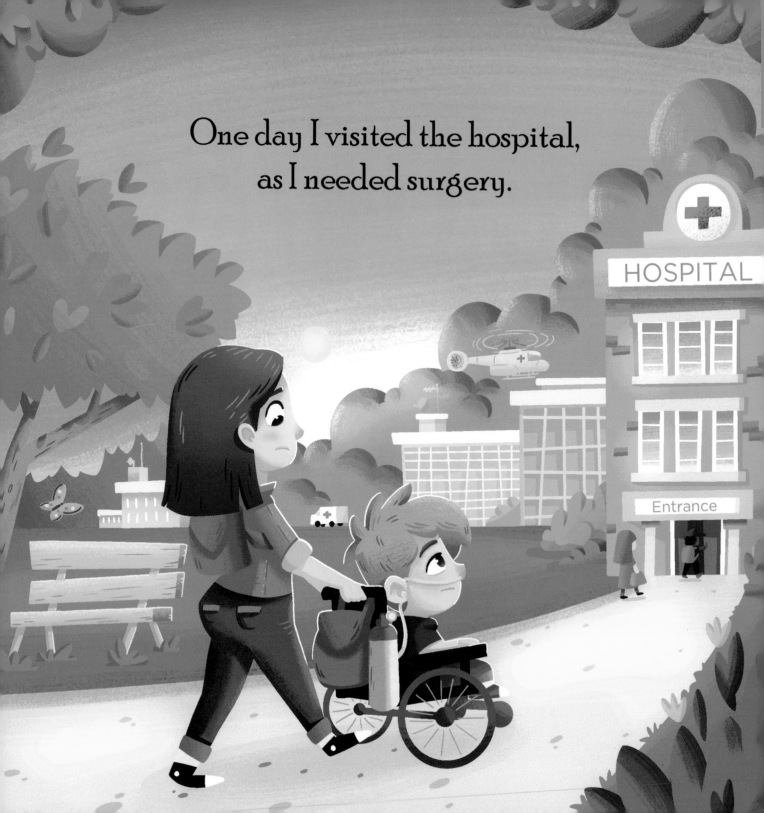

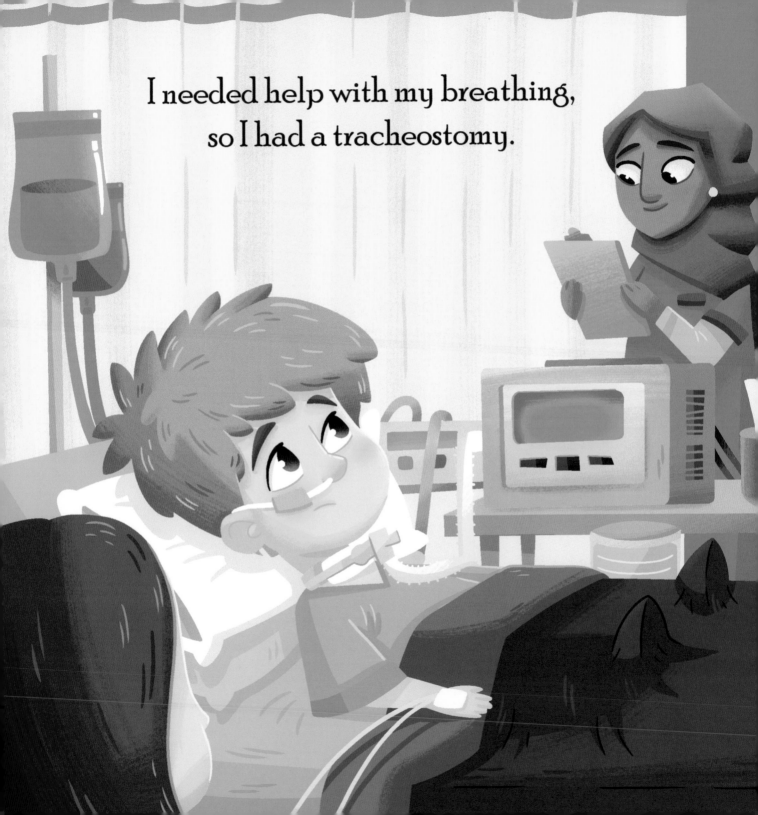

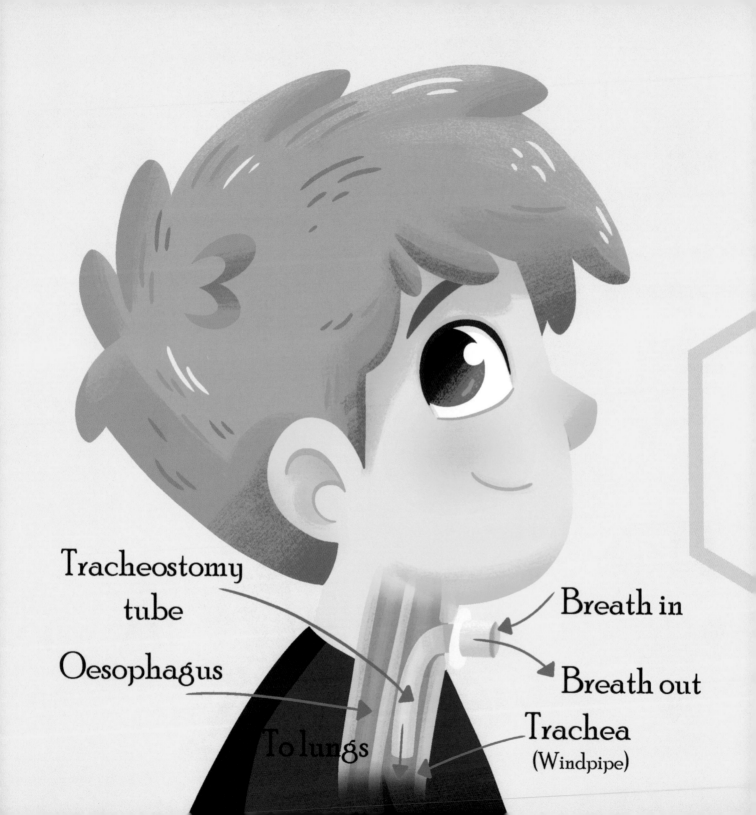

Tracheostomy tube

Oesophagus

To lungs

Breath in

Breath out

Trachea
(Windpipe)

A hole was made into my neck
and then a tube went in.
It opened up my windpipe,
which helped me breathe again.

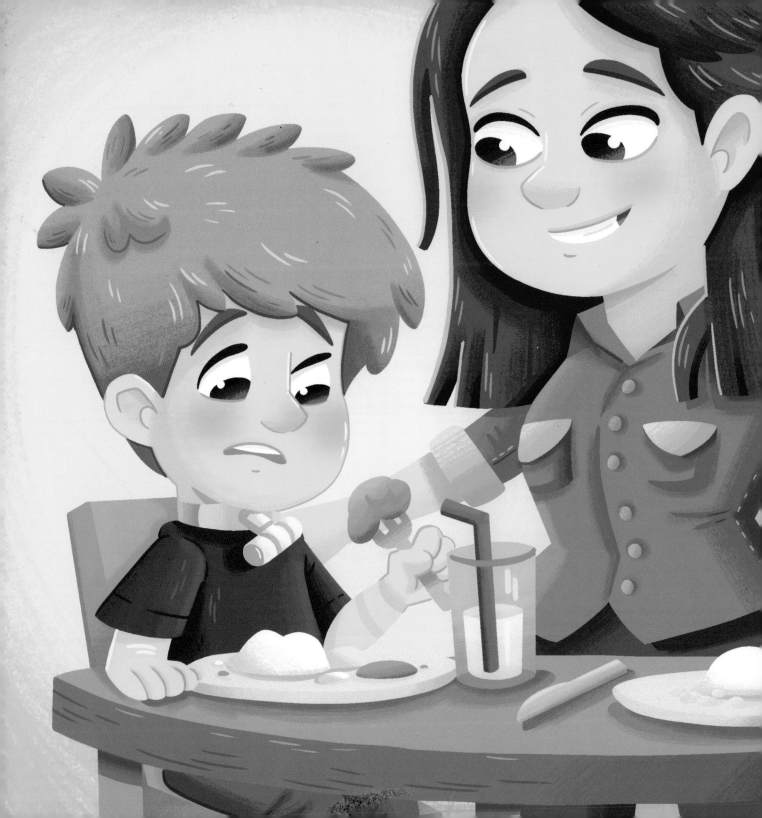

After having my surgery,
it was hard to swallow and eat.
I also found it hard to talk,
so I had speech therapy.

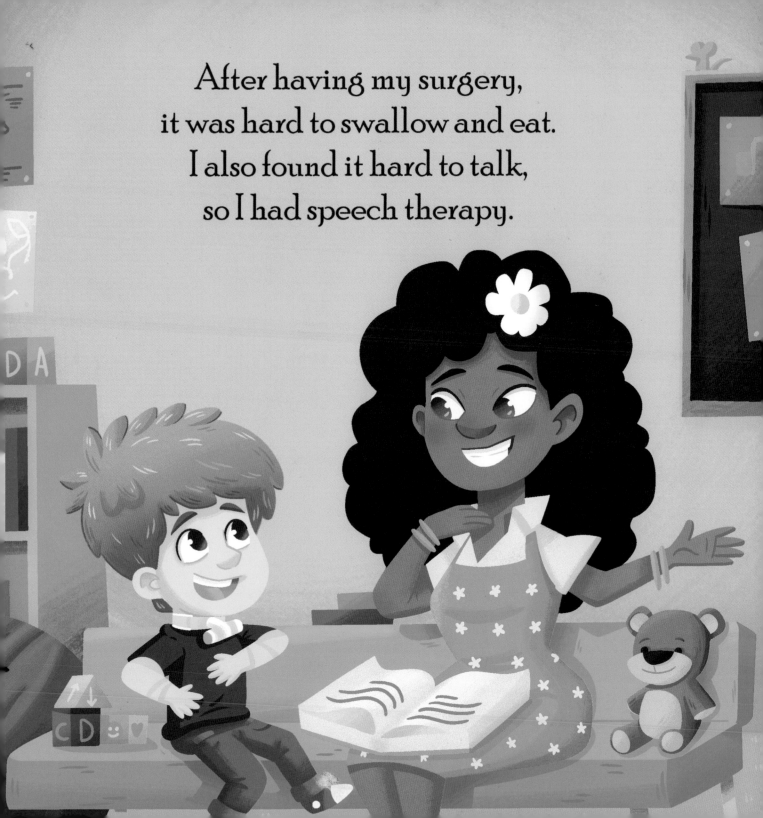

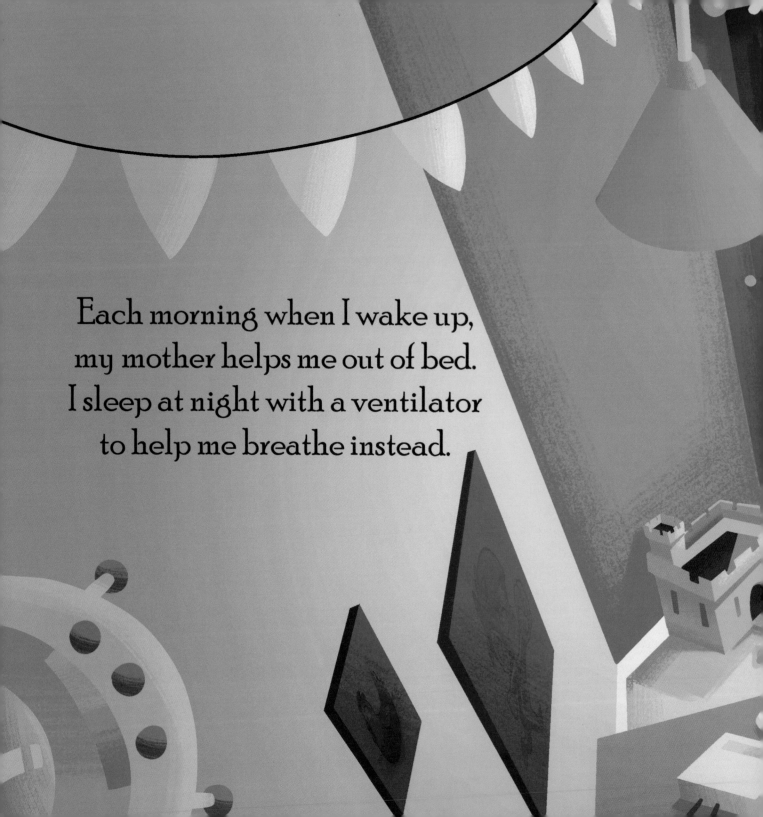

Each morning when I wake up,
my mother helps me out of bed.
I sleep at night with a ventilator
to help me breathe instead.

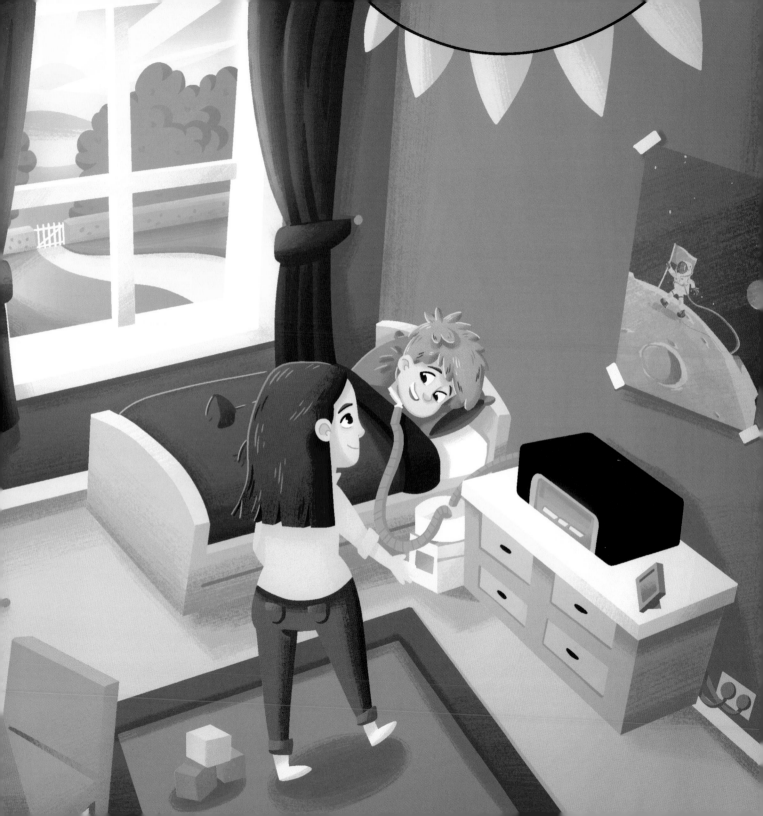

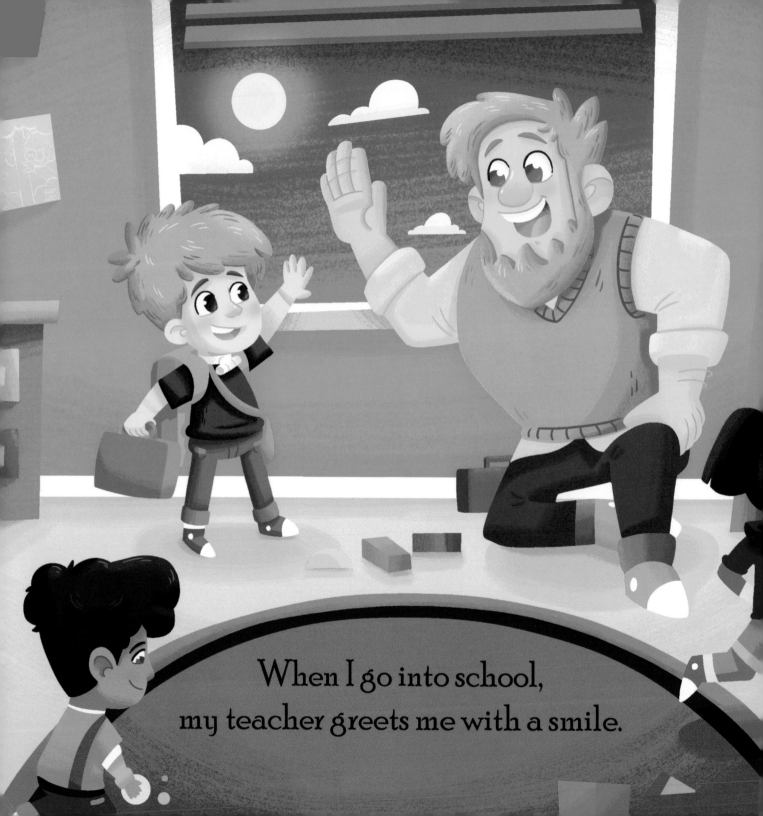

When I go into school,
my teacher greets me with a smile.

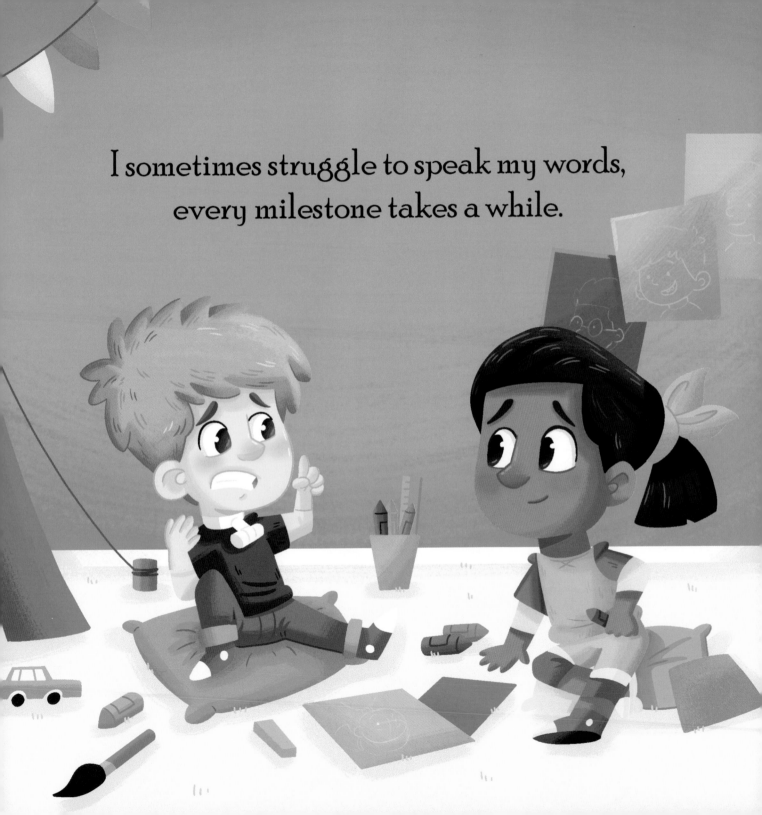

I sometimes struggle to speak my words,
every milestone takes a while.

There are so many things that I can do,
when I have my support.
I really like to sing and dance
and play tennis on the court.

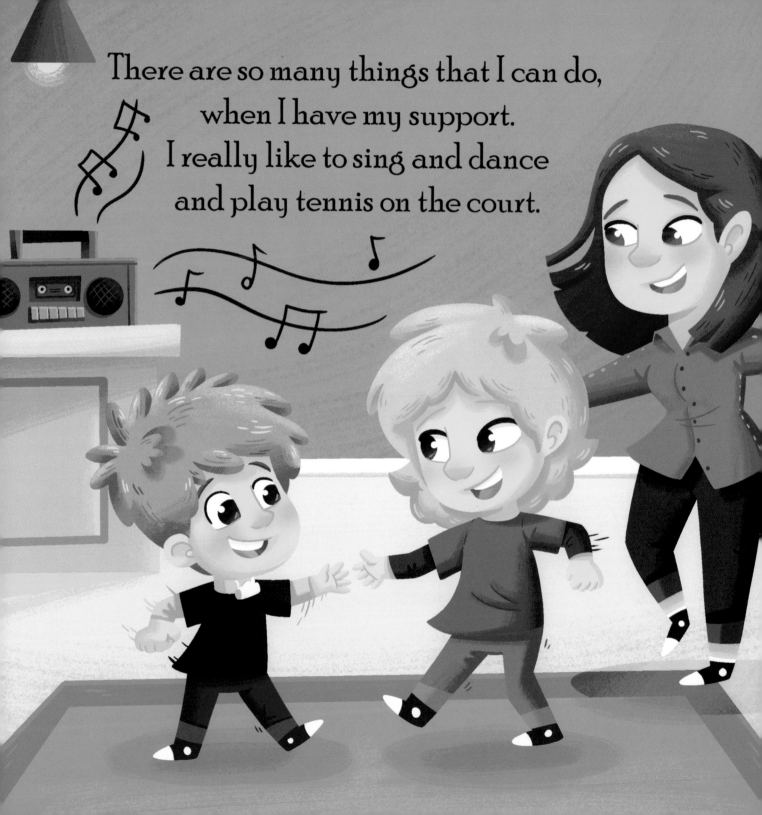

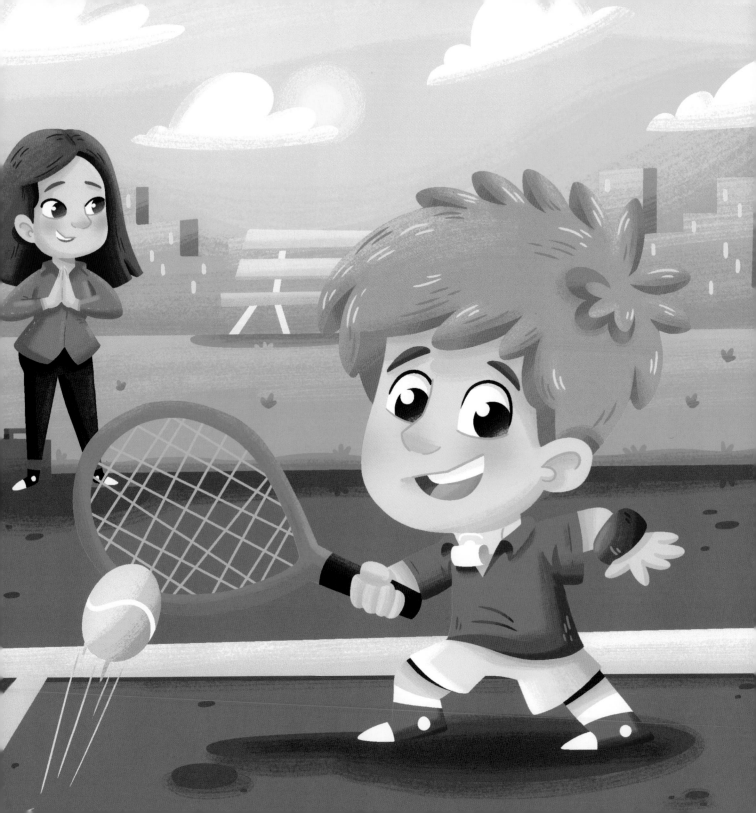

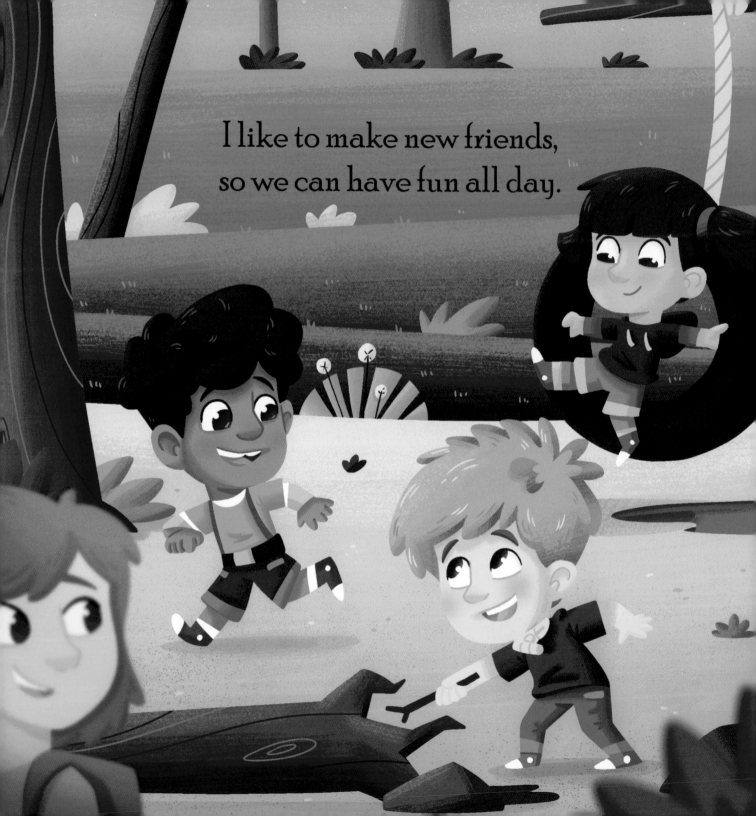

I like to make new friends,
so we can have fun all day.

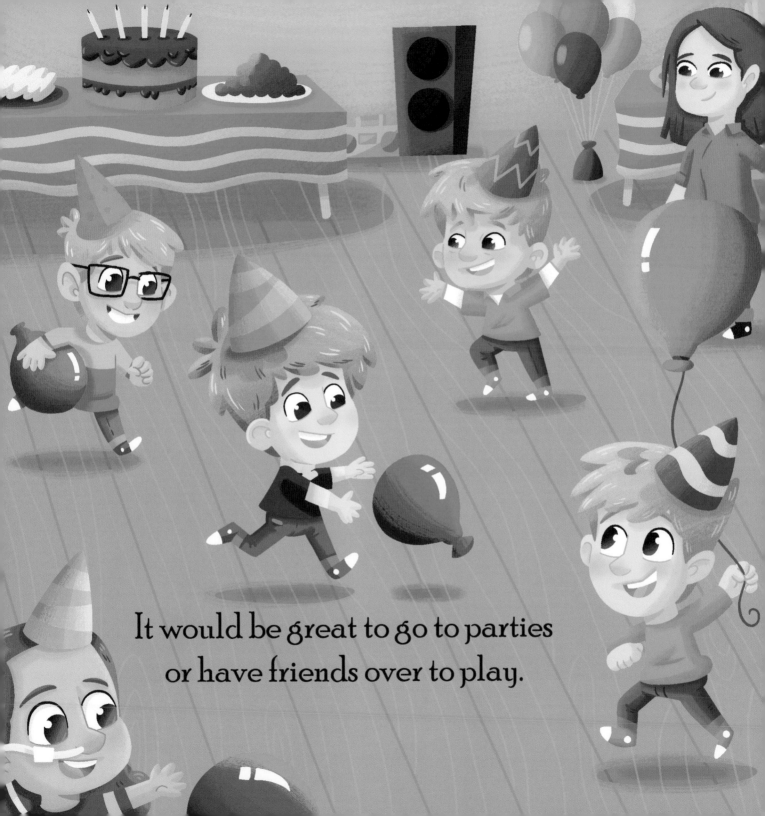

It would be great to go to parties
or have friends over to play.

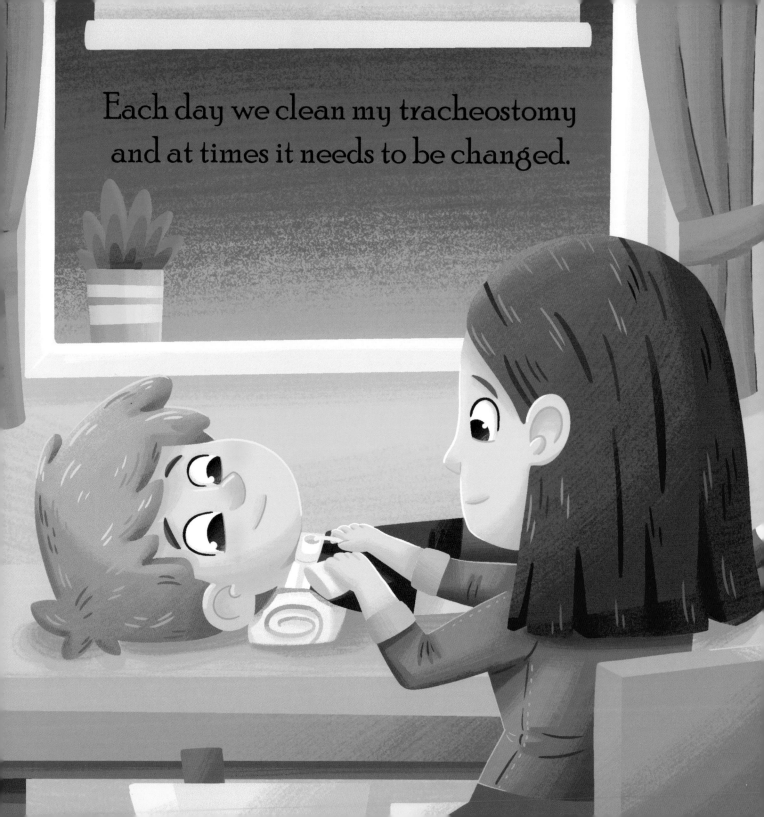

Each day we clean my tracheostomy and at times it needs to be changed.

This keeps me nice and healthy,
with the supplies nicely arranged.

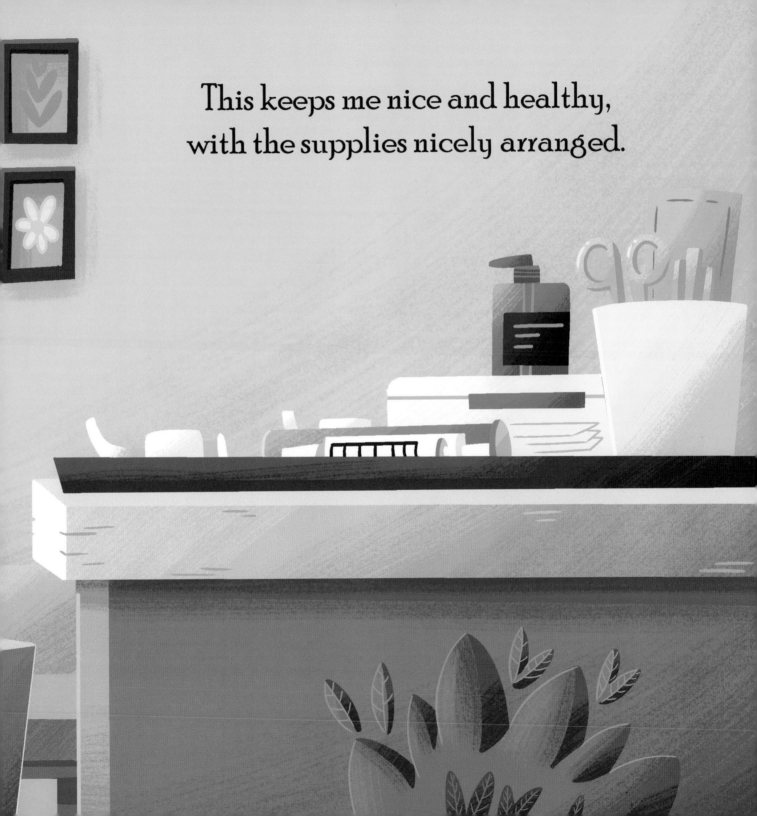

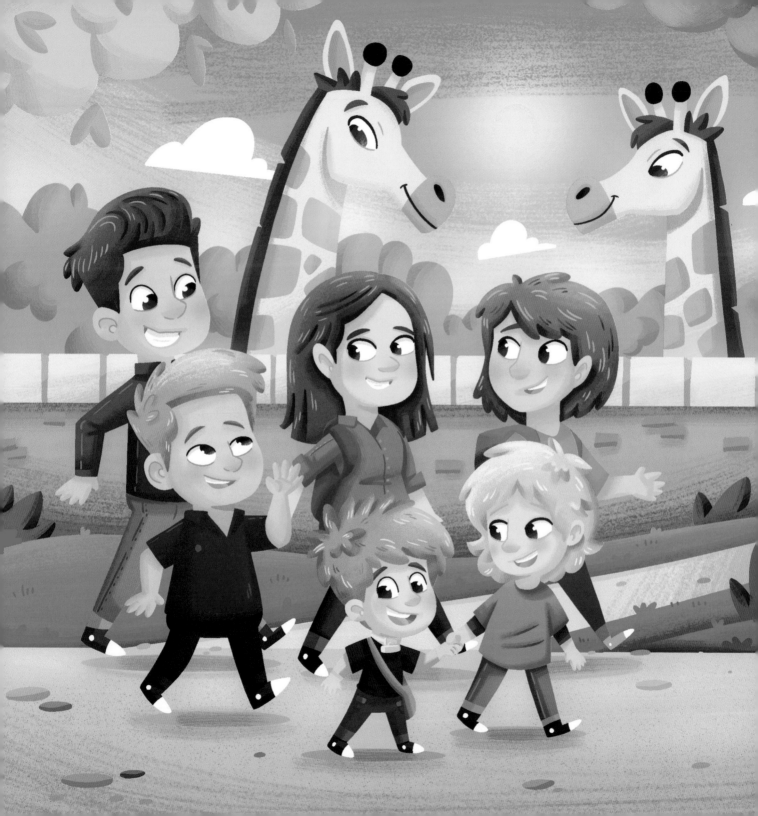

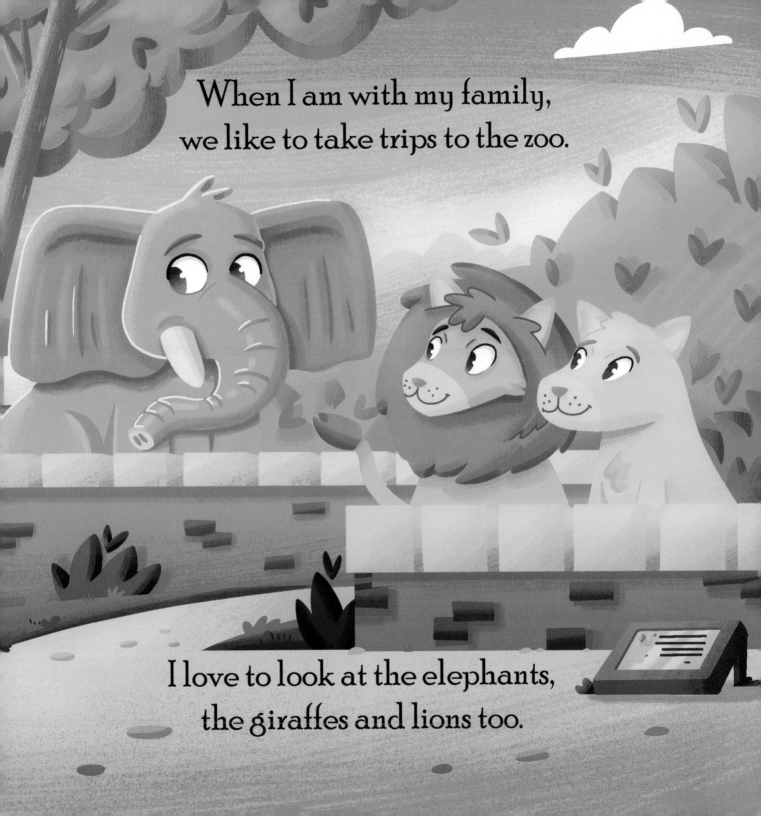

When I am with my family,
we like to take trips to the zoo.

I love to look at the elephants,
the giraffes and lions too.

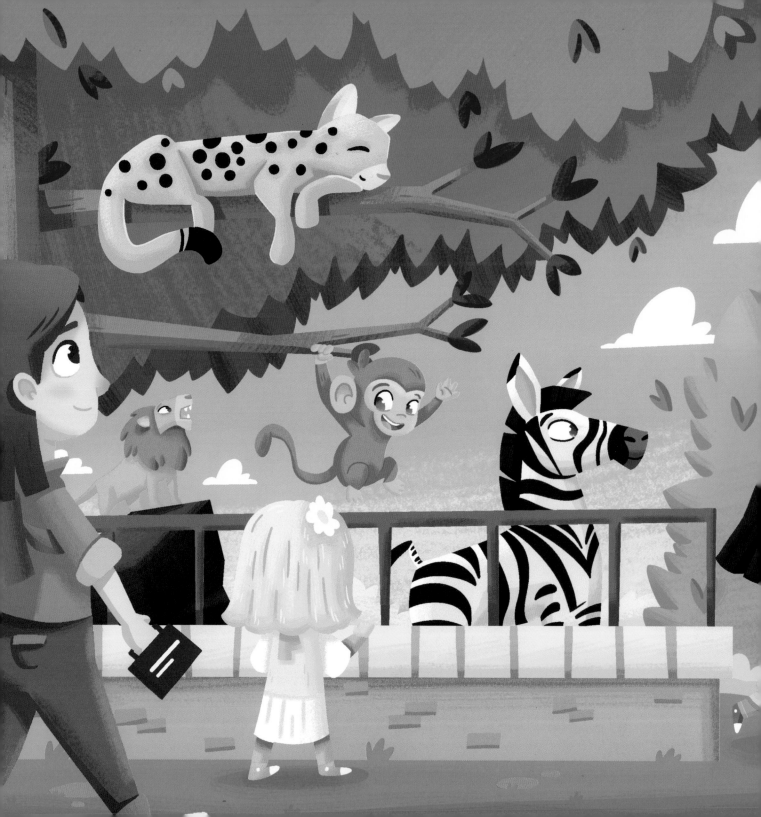

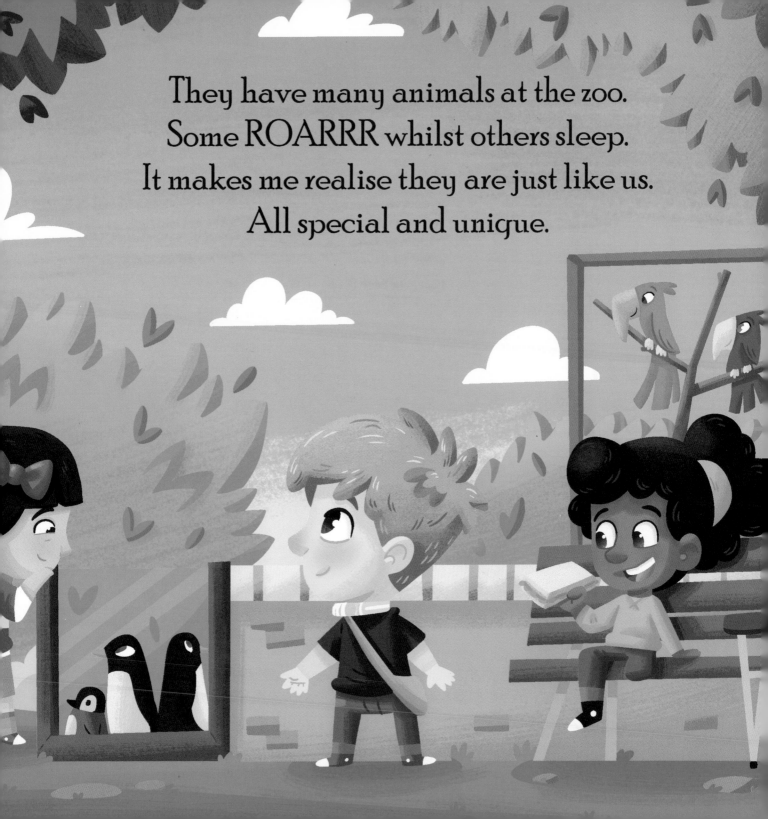

They have many animals at the zoo.
Some ROARRR whilst others sleep.
It makes me realise they are just like us.
All special and unique.

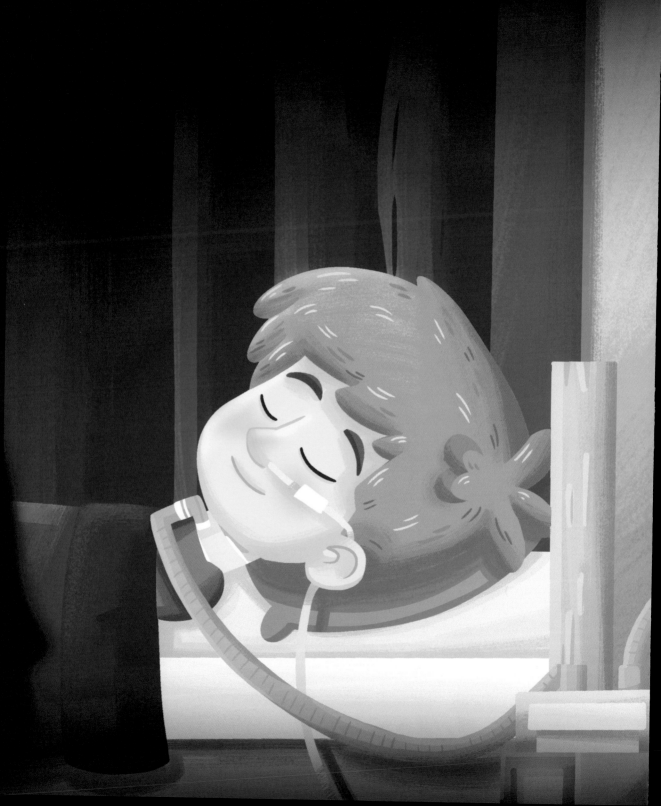

At the end of the day when the sun goes down,
I feel tired and get undressed.
I lay in bed with my ventilator,
which helps me breathe and rest.

So now you know about my Tracheostomy
and the things I can do.
Let's be friends and please tell me,
what abilities are in you?

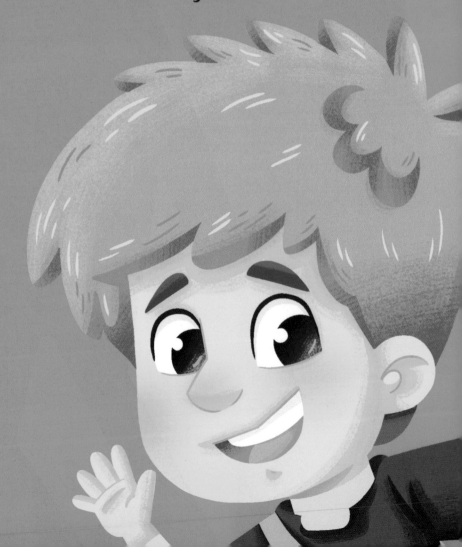

Write down your *super* abilities:

_____

_____

_____

_____

What makes you happy?
Please draw below.

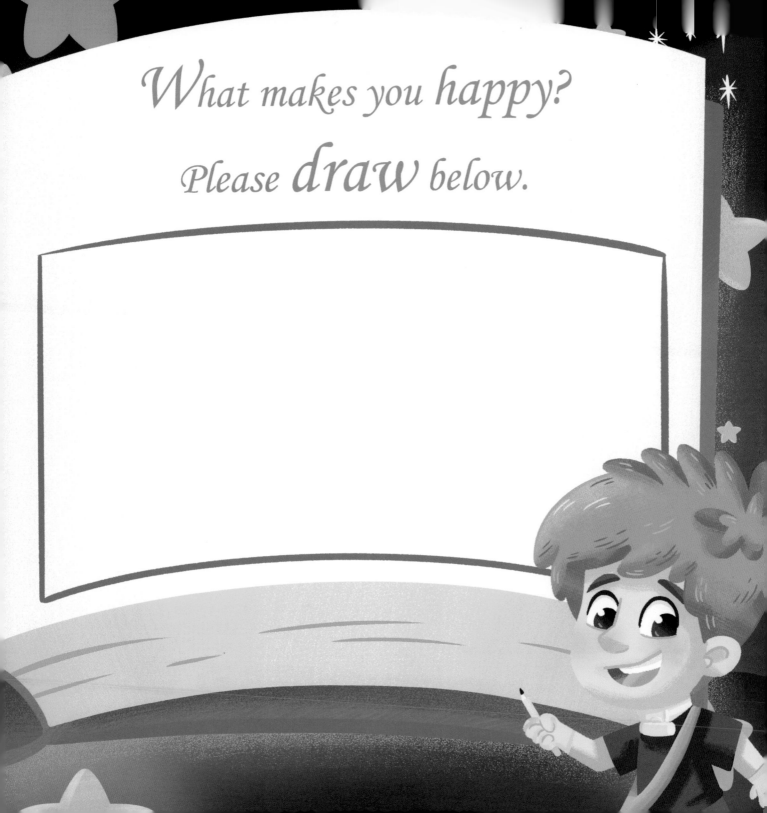

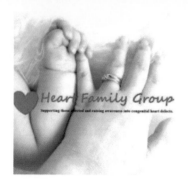

Heart Family Group founded in the UK in 2014.

We support families with congenital heart defects.
We have a public Facebook page and a private group for families.

We donate each year around Christmas time to cardiac wards and we arrange events for families to meet in person.

Our aim is to provide support each day of the year.

This group is run by families themselves who have children with congenital heart defects.

  /HeartFamilyGroup

  /groups/MurrishHeartFamily

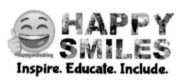

Happy Smiles was initially created as a blog, inspired by a young man with complex needs who always has a smile on his face!
They empower young adults with various additional and complex needs, to deliver inclusive training workshops to schools, community groups, charities and more!

Call - 07917221503

Email - info@happysmilesblog.co.uk

Website - www.happysmilesblog.co.uk

  /happysmilesblog

  @happysmilesblog

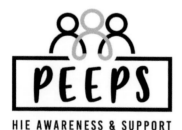

We support those affected by HIE (hypoxic-ischaemic encephalopathy), and raise awareness.

Email: info@peeps-hie.org

Website: www.peeps-hie.org

  /peeps.hie

  @PeepsHIE

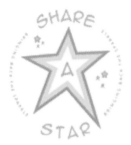

Share a Star helps seriously unwell children and teenagers through supporting the whole family.

We create handmade bespoke holding stars for the youngster to hold onto and each one is unique to the child. In that star, it has their world in it.
We've made such a variety of stars from Ariana Grande to Foxy Bingo!
We support the siblings as well through some of our many projects.
We send out happy boxes, and send some of our stars on special outings.
We also run a project called Forever a Star, to support families through the first stage of bereavement.

Website - www.shareastar.org

Email - Info@shareastar.org.uk

  /ShareAStarCharity

@shareastarcharity

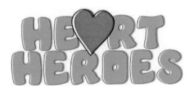

Heart Heroes supports families of children living with congenital heart disease and heart problems.

Our goal is for children and their siblings to be included in all our events, along with parents, grandparents, aunties, uncles and any other close family.

Our charity is run solely by volunteers and we are always looking for additional support.

email@heartheroes.co.uk

Website: www.heartheroes.co.uk

 /heartheroesglos

 @HeartHeroes1

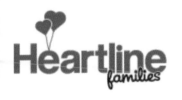

Heartline supports children with heart disorders and their families, whatever the condition, wherever it is treated.

Website: www.heartline.org.uk

 /HeartlineUK

 @heartlineuk

About the Author

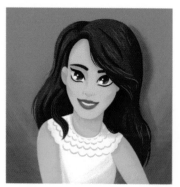

My name is Gemma Keir, I am the book author for "The abilities in me" children's book series from Hertfordshire, England. I am a mum to a child with a range of medical conditions, including 22q Deletion who has inspired me to write these incredible stories. I am proud to have received qualifications in Special Educational Needs and Disabilities and Sensory Awareness plus specialist training in Behaviour and Safeguarding. These books provide awareness of a range of needs in children today and will be extremely popular for school settings and families who have a child with these conditions. I aim to change the whole perception of these children by promoting the abilities they do have and prevent potential bullying later in that child's life. I feel that this is possible, because children around them will be taught, from a young age and in a positive light, to have awareness and be open-minded. My vision is for children with special educational needs and disabilities to have a book to read about a character who is just like them. I aim to bring inclusivity to children's literature, acceptance and positivity.

www.theabilitiesinme.com

www.facebook.com/theabilitiesinmebookseries

About the Illustrator

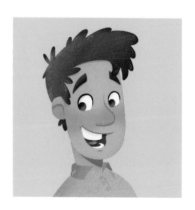

My name is Adam Walker-Parker, I am a professional illustrator from Scotland. I have worked in the art industry for 12 years now, I began my career as an artist, choosing to paint figurative and wildlife paintings.
I now illustrate children's books and find joy in creating something magical and inspiring for children to see.

www.awalkerparker.com

www.facebook.com/awalkerparkerillustration

www.instagram.com/awalkerparkerillustration

MORE BOOKS COMING SOON

We create children's picture books, based on characters of young children with varying disabilities.
Each book will feature a child with a condition, and we aim to create a bright, colourful and positive outlook on
every child with special needs. We are all unique and beautiful in every way, shape and form. This collection of
books will show how each child can celebrate their abilities within their disability, find acceptance and create
awareness to those around them. These books will touch the hearts of your homes, schools and hospital settings,
and most importantly, your child will have a book to read, based on a special character, just like them.

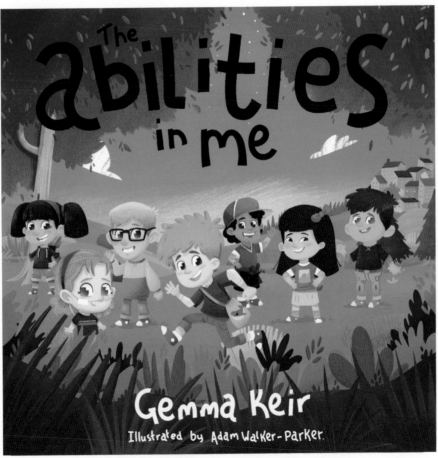

Title: The Abilities In Me - Children's Book Series
Written by Gemma Keir
Cover and Illustrations by Adam Walker-Parker

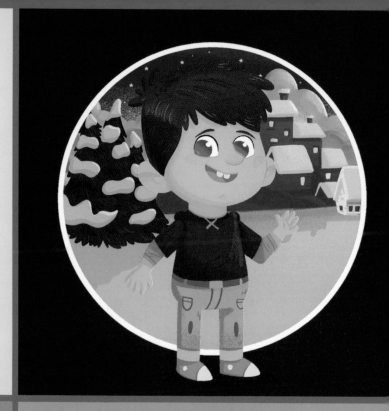

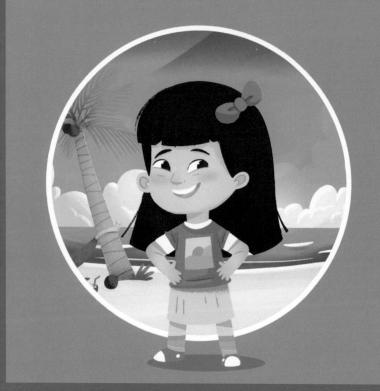

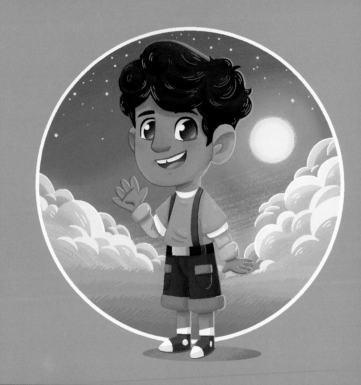

Printed in Great Britain
by Amazon

40734683R00021